Unknown

Mitchell Holloway

1. Starlight's Song

Beneath the sky, where stars belong,
The universe hums its timeless song.
Each flickering light, a whispered plea,
Echoes of love in eternity.

2. Petals of Time

Roses bloom, then fall away,
Caught in the tides of fleeting days.
Yet in the soil, their seeds will sow,
A timeless promise: life will grow.

3. Shadows and Suns

Where shadows stretch, the sun will rise,
Casting light on hidden skies.
Even in darkness, embers gleam,
Dreams still stir within the dream.

4. Whispers of the Forest

In the woods, where silence reigns,
Each leaf a story, each breeze explains.
The earth speaks softly, roots run deep,
A cradle of whispers where secrets sleep.

5. A Stranger's Smile

A fleeting glance, a spark, a pause,
A smile born with no known cause.
In that moment, the world stood still,
A stranger's warmth, a gentle thrill.

6. Moonlit Waves

The sea reflects a silver light,
Waves that dance beneath the night.

A lullaby sung to restless souls,
Binding hearts to ocean shoals.

7. Echoes of Yesterday

The clock ticks softly; time moves slow,
A haunting dance where memories go.
Each fleeting shadow, a fleeting sigh,
Echoes of years that drift and die.

8. Wildflower Dreams

Amidst the weeds, wildflowers grew,
Bright and bold, kissed by dew.
They whispered tales to the passing breeze,
Of freedom found beyond the trees.

9. The Silent Flame

A candle burns, its light subdued,
A quiet fire, a steady mood.
Its flame may falter, flicker, sway,
But steadfastly, it lights the way.

10. The Wanderer's Wish

Oh, to roam where skies are wide,
To feel the earth, no walls to confide.
The wind, my guide; the stars, my map,
Freedom flows in every gap.

11. The River's Secret

Flowing soft, through rock and stone,
The river sings, yet walks alone.
Its melody, a tale untold,

Of ancient dreams and treasures bold.

12. A Single Feather

Drifting down, from skies unknown,
A feather falls, soft as a tone.
A message carried, light as air,
Of freedom found, and hearts laid bare.

13. Lantern Glow

Through mist and dusk, the lantern glows,
A golden thread the darkness knows.
Its flame, though small, burns bright and true,
A beacon strong for those who knew.

14. The Forgotten Garden

Behind the walls, past gates of rust,
A garden thrives beneath the dust.
Flowers bloom in secret shade,
A quiet realm by time betrayed.

15. Wind's Embrace

The wind it speaks, in tones so low,
It wraps around, then lets you go.
A fleeting friend, a lover wild,
Its touch both fierce and soft as a child.

16. Threads of Gold

The loom of fate weaves threads unseen,
A pattern vast, both cruel and keen.
Yet here and there, a golden thread,
Reminds us life is richly fed.

17. Winter's Silence

The snow descends, a quiet grace,

It softens time, and slows the race.
In winter's silence, hearts may heal,
Beneath the frost, the earth is real.

18. The Broken Clock

The clock stood still, its hands at rest,
No longer marking time's unrest.
And yet, the world continued on,
As if the ticking was never gone.

19. Star-Crossed Shores

Across the waves, two shores collide,
Bound by dreams and oceans wide.
Though far apart, their love still grows,
A tether strong as the tide that flows.

20. The Last Ember

A fire dwindles, its light grows faint,
Yet in the ash lies no constraint.
For from the ember, warmth will spread,
And kindled hearts will rise instead.

1. The Weeping Willow

Beneath the willow, where shadows play,
The world grows soft at the close of day.
Her branches droop, her whispers low,
A gentle hymn to those who know.

She saw the lovers who once did meet,
Beneath her boughs, where time is sweet.
Their vows were spoken, their hearts laid bare,
In the fragrant touch of summer air.

But seasons turned, and leaves would fall,
The willow watched through it all.
Her roots sank deep where secrets lay,
Stories forgotten, lost to decay.

Now she stands, an ancient queen,
Guarding dreams that might have been.
Her song is soft, her tears still flow,
For time moves on, yet she won't go.

2. Ballad of the Desert Rose

In the desert where the sun lays claim,
And sands burn bright like a golden flame,
There blooms a rose, fierce and wild,
A flower born of the earth's exile.

Her petals crimson, her leaves jade green,
A beauty harsh, yet serene.
Her roots drink deep from hidden streams,
A life sustained by quiet dreams.

Travelers pass, with weary eyes,
And see her there beneath the skies.
A single bloom in endless sand,
A miracle wrought by nature's hand.

But none can pluck her, none can claim,
For the desert rose plays no man's game.
She is a symbol, a quiet lore,
Of resilience found on barren shores.

3. The Lighthouse Keeper

Alone he stands, the keeper of light,
Guiding ships through the perilous night.
His tower tall, a beacon true,
A guardian's task, his sacred view.

The storms they howl, the waves they crash,
Against the rocks with a vengeful lash.
Yet still he tends the flame so bright,
A solitary warrior in the fight.

His days are long, his words are few,
The ocean his master, forever anew.
He watches tides and fading stars,
Dreaming of lands that lie afar.

Though lonely, he finds solace still,
In the light he guards with iron will.
For every ship that safely steers,
He whispers a prayer, quiet with tears.

4. Forest of Forgotten Kings

Deep in the forest, where no paths lead,
Lie ruins hidden by vine and weed.
Once mighty thrones of marble white,
Now crumble beneath the moon's pale light.

The trees have grown where halls once stood,
Their roots entwined with ancient wood.
And whispers linger, carried by breeze,
Of kings who knelt to time's decrees.

The forest hums with secrets lost,
Of battles fought and lives the cost.
Yet peace now reigns where swords once clashed,
And nature heals what greed had dashed.

So tread with care, for the earth still sings,
In the sacred realm of forgotten kings.

5. The Storm's Serenade

The storm it comes with thunder's roar,
A tempest wild that shakes the shore.

Its winds they wail, its rains they cry,
A symphony played in the weeping sky.

The trees they bend, the rivers swell,
Nature's fury, a tale to tell.
Yet in the chaos, a beauty lies,
A dance of elements beneath dark skies.

For storms must come to cleanse the air,
To bring the earth a love so rare.
And when it fades, the world is new,
Refreshed by rain, bathed in dew.

6. The Wanderer's Anthem

I walk the roads that none have named,
Through lands unknown, untamed, unclaimed.
With stars my guide, and winds my friend,
I seek the paths that never end.

The mountains call, their echoes deep,
Their peaks a promise I must keep.
The rivers sing, their waters glide,
A siren's tune I cannot bide.

I am the wanderer, ever free,
A soul unbound, a restless sea.
No hearth, no home, no ties to bind,
Just endless horizons to find.

7. Song of the Winter's Heart

Winter's breath is cold and clear,
It whispers close, it draws you near.
The snow it falls, a quiet shroud,
A blanket soft, both pale and proud.

The trees stand bare, their branches thin,
Their slumber deep, their dreams within.

The rivers freeze, their voices stilled,
Their icy veins with silence filled.

Yet winter's heart is not of gloom,
It holds a peace that flowers bloom.
For in its stillness, life prepares,
To burst anew when spring declares.

craft each poem with care. Let's start! □

1. The Eternal Flame

Beneath the stars where shadows creep,
A fire burns while the world sleeps.
Its light is soft, yet fierce and bright,
A beacon strong in the endless night.

The flame remembers times long gone,
When kings would rise and wars were won.
It flickered through the ages past,
A steadfast glow, a flame to last.

Its embers speak in quiet tones,
Of ancient hands and polished stones.
They built this pyre, they fed its glow,
A symbol strong of all they'd know.

And though the winds may howl and wail,
The fire endures; it will not fail.
For in its heart, a truth is found:
That hope can rise where ashes mound.

2. A World in the Raindrop

A single drop falls from the sky,
A tiny world to the passerby.

It holds reflections, both vast and small,
A fleeting glimpse of the all-in-all.

Within its curve, the heavens bend,
A universe with no known end.
Mountains stand in miniature grace,
Clouds drift slow in its fragile space.

Yet soon it lands, and then it fades,
Into the earth, where life pervades.
Its journey brief, its purpose clear,
To nourish life, to disappear.

Oh, tiny drop, so full, so free,
A fleeting mirror of eternity.

3. The Last Oak

On a hill where winds do roam,
Stands an oak, both vast and alone.
Its roots run deep, its branches high,
A bridge between the earth and sky.

The seasons pass, its leaves will fall,
But still it towers, proud and tall.
Through summer heat and winter snow,
Its wisdom lingers, its strength will show.

For countless years, it's watched the land,
From farmers' toil to nature's hand.
Yet now it waits, as silence grows,
The final witness of what it knows.

And when it falls, as all things must,
Its trunk will crumble, return to dust.
But in its place, new life will spring,
A cycle endless, a song to sing.

4. A Song for the Stars

Sing, O stars, in the velvet sky,
Whisper songs to the wondering eye.
Tell of ages when the earth was new,
When time was young, and so were you.

Shine, O stars, with your ancient light,
Guide the lost through the darkest night.
Each twinkle holds a memory vast,
A glimpse of futures, a hint of past.

Though you are far, your voices near,
A chorus grand that all can hear.
And even when your light will fade,
Your songs will linger, a serenade.

So sing, O stars, your timeless tune,
For hearts will listen beneath the moon.

5. The River's Refrain

Through forest green and valleys wide,
The river flows, a gentle guide.
Its voice is soft, yet full of might,
A constant hymn through day and night.

It carries whispers of mountain springs,
Of soaring birds and their fleeting wings.
It knows the tales of fish and stone,
Of ancient roots and seeds once sown.

The river bends, the river turns,
It cools the earth where sunlight burns.
Yet to the sea, it always goes,
Where waves embrace and the ocean flows.

Oh, river wild, your path runs true,
A mirror bright of skies so blue.

6. A Lover's Lament

Beneath the willow, where shadows weep,
I laid my heart for love to keep.
But time is cruel, and fate unkind,
It steals the joy and leaves the blind.

Your touch was soft as morning dew,
Your words a song I never knew.
Yet now I stand where silence reigns,
A heart once whole, now wrapped in chains.

The stars above still gleam so bright,
But none can heal this endless night.
For love was mine, but love is gone,
A fleeting spark before the dawn.

Oh, willow tree, please guard my soul,
And keep my love, now ashes cold.

7. The Mountain Speaks

High above where eagles soar,
The mountain stands, a timeless lore.
Its cliffs are steep, its peaks are bare,
Yet beauty lingers everywhere.

It speaks in winds, in echoes vast,
Of glaciers gone and ages past.
Its stones hold secrets, carved by time,
In jagged peaks and slopes that climb.

The mountain calls to hearts so brave,
To those who seek what cannot cave.
For though its heights seem far and wide,
It holds the dreams that we confide.

So climb, O soul, to heights unseen,
And touch the clouds where life feels clean.

8. A Field of Gold

The wheat it sways beneath the sun,
A golden dance where life's begun.
Each stalk a tale, each seed a dream,
Of labor's hand and nature's scheme.

The farmer walks, his steps are slow,
Through fields that spark, through seeds that grow.
He knows the soil, the earth's embrace,
The joy of harvest, the toil of grace.

And when the day gives way to night,
The stars above will cast their light.
A field of gold, both vast and true,
A testament to the old and new.

9. The Cave of Wonders

Deep in the earth, where darkness dwells,
There lies a cave with hidden spells.
Its walls are lined with gems that gleam,
A treasure trove, a dreamer's dream.

The air is cold, the silence deep,
A sacred place where secrets sleep.
The stalactites drip, the echoes call,
A haunting tune within the hall.

But tread with care, for shadows wake,
And treasure comes with risks to take.
For in the cave where wonders glow,
The heart must choose which path to go.

10. The Edge of the World

At the edge of the world, where the oceans fall,
There lies a place that beckons all.
Its skies are vast, its winds untamed,
Its beauty raw, its power unnamed.

The cliffs they stand, both proud and bold,
A final guard to the stories told.
The waves below, they crash and roar,
A siren's cry to the distant shore.

And those who stand at the world's great end,
Will find no foe, no need to mend.
For in the vastness, the truth is clear:
The edge is simply the start from here.

11. The Phoenix's Cry

From ashes gray, the phoenix soars,
A blaze of fire, a life restored.
Its feathers burn with crimson hue,
A testament to life renewed.

Through pain it rises, through flames it grows,
A creature born where endings close.
The skies it claims, the earth it leaves,
A fiery trail through which it weaves.

Its song is fierce, a mournful tone,
Of lives rebuilt and seeds once sown.
And though it fades, it knows the truth:
From every end, there comes new youth.

12. The Meadow's Prayer

The meadow lies in quiet bloom,
Beneath the sun, beneath the moon.
Its grasses hum, its flowers sigh,
A whispered prayer to the open sky.

The bees they hum, the breeze it sways,
Through endless nights and golden days.
Each petal soft, each stem so true,
A tapestry of green and blue.

But hidden deep, where roots entwine,
The meadow guards a sacred shrine.
Its soil is rich with dreams untold,
Of life and love, a heart of gold.

13. The Hunter's Shadow

Through forests dark, the hunter goes,
His bow in hand, his steps are slow.
The moonlight falls, the shadows creep,
Through whispered woods where secrets sleep.

He tracks his prey with eyes so keen,
Through thorny brush and leaves of green.
But in the silence, his heart does wane,
For in the hunt, he feels the pain.

The woods are wild, their call is strong,
A haunting tune, a hunter's song.
And though he walks with purpose clear,
The hunter's shadow hides his fear.

14. The Bridge of Stars

There is a bridge that none can see,
It spans the sky, it crosses the sea.
Its arches gleam with starlight bright,
A pathway built of endless night.

The weary tread its quiet span,
Each step a wish, each dream a plan.
It leads them home, it sets them free,
A bridge between eternity.

Though fleeting, it will always shine,
A gift from stars, a grand design.
For in its glow, all hearts will find,
A thread that binds both space and time.

15. The Clockmaker's Dream

The clockmaker sits in his shadowed shop,
Where ticking fills each silent stop.
His hands are steady, his tools precise,
Creating moments, both bold and nice.

Each gear he turns, each spring he winds,
A world of time within confined.
And though his craft is truly grand,
He dreams of time he cannot command.

For hours pass, and years will fade,
A truth no clock has ever swayed.
Yet in his dream, he finds his art:
A ticking rhythm, a beating heart.

16. The Lantern Bearer

Through mist and fog, the lantern glows,
A golden flame where darkness grows.
The bearer walks, their path unknown,
Through haunted woods, through lands alone.

Their steps are light, their spirit strong,
Their flame a guide, their will a song.
And though the night is vast and cold,
The lantern burns with stories told.

For every shadow hides a face,
And every fear, a hidden grace.
The bearer knows, though dark the land,
The light will rise where courage stands.

17. The Sorcerer's Tower

High on a cliff where the winds collide,
A tower stands, where shadows hide.
Its walls are etched with runes of old,

A fortress strong, both dark and cold.

The sorcerer dwells in his lonely keep,
Where books of magic in silence sleep.
His spells are whispers, his power vast,
A relic born of ages past.

Yet in his heart, a hollow lies,
A longing deep, beneath the skies.
For though his magic bends the land,
It cannot touch the mortal hand.

18. The Ocean's Lament

The ocean sings a mournful tune,
Beneath the sun, beneath the moon.
Its waves they rise, its tides they fall,
A symphony that touches all.

It speaks of ships, now lost and gone,
Of sailors' cries and morning dawns.
It tells of shores both near and far,
Of endless dreams beneath the stars.

Yet in its depth, its heart does ache,
For every gift, there's much to take.
The ocean's beauty hides its pain,
A timeless grief within its chain.

19. The Path Untaken

There lies a path, both dark and bright,
It twists through shadow, it bends to light.
Its stones are smooth, its trails are clear,
Yet none will tread for they know fear.

For on this path, the soul must bare,
Its truest self, its deepest care.
No lies can linger, no mask can stay,

For every truth will find its way.

Yet those who walk, though hearts may quake,
Will find a joy that none can fake.
For on this path, where courage reigns,
The truest freedom breaks its chains.

20. The Forest's Heartbeat

Deep in the woods where the wild things grow,
A heartbeat hums, a steady flow.
The trees they sway, the roots they sing,
A rhythm born of everything.

The fox it dances, the deer it leaps,
The owl it watches, the wolf it keeps.
The forest breathes with life unseen,
A world untouched, a realm serene.

Yet in its heart, a warning cries,
Of fallen trees and broken skies.
The forest pleads, it calls to all,
To save its soul before it falls.

26. The Warrior's Oath

With sword in hand and heart so true,
The warrior steps where few would pursue.
Their path is dark, their trials vast,
A journey carved by the shadows cast.

Through fields of battle, through cries of pain,
They seek no glory, they seek no gain.
For every strike, a vow they keep,
To guard the weak, the lost, the meek.

Though scars may line their weathered skin,

Their soul remains a light within.
And when the fight at last is done,
Their story shines beneath the sun.

27. A Garden in the Rain

The rain it falls on leaves so green,
A gentle mist, a quiet scene.
Each droplet sings, each petal sways,
A melody born of silvered days.

The roses bloom, their colors bright,
A beacon bold in the fading light.
The daisies dance, the ivy grows,
Through every storm, the garden knows.

For rain is life, a gift profound,
A blessing poured upon the ground.
And in its wake, the garden thrives,
A living song where love survives.

28. The Ghost's Lament

In moonlit halls where silence reigns,
The ghost walks soft, bound by chains.
Their whispers drift, a mournful sound,
A cry for peace they've never found.

They linger long in shadows deep,
A restless soul that cannot sleep.
Their memories fade, their voice grows thin,
A shadow lost to the world within.

And yet they yearn, their heart still burns,
For love they lost, for time that turns.
Oh, grant them rest, a final peace,
And let their sorrow at last release.

29. The Star-Maker

In the void where silence flows,
The star-maker works, and galaxies grow.
Their hands of light, their breath a flame,
They shape the heavens, they forge the frame.

Each star they place, a jewel so bright,
A tiny sun in the endless night.
Their canvas vast, their brush divine,
A masterpiece in every line.

And though unseen by mortal eyes,
Their work endures in the endless skies.
For every star that gleams above,
Is born of labor, is born of love.

30. The Bell at Dawn

The bell it rings as dawn breaks clear,
A golden chime for all to hear.
Its echo rolls through fields and trees,
A call that dances upon the breeze.

It speaks of hope, it sings of peace,
A herald bright for night's release.
And those who hear its gentle tone,
Will find their hearts no longer alone.

Oh, bell of dawn, so pure, so true,
Your song reminds the world anew.
That every day, no matter how long,
Begins again with a hopeful song.

31. The Eternal Library

In hidden halls where whispers grow,
A library vast, a sacred glow.
Its shelves stretch high, its books untold,
A treasure trove of wisdom old.

The words they hum, the pages sigh,
Each book a world where dreams can fly.
And those who seek its hallowed lore,
Will find a key to every door.

Yet tread with care, for knowledge deep,
Can stir the heart or make it weep.
The library waits, a timeless friend,
A haven true where journeys end.

32. The Stonecutter's Song

The stonecutter works with steady hand,
Carving dreams from the solid land.
Each strike of steel, each chisel's kiss,
Brings forth a form, a shape of bliss.

The marble yields, the granite bends,
To artistry that never ends.
Their work is slow, yet bold and grand,
A masterpiece from grains of sand.

And though their name may fade with years,
Their legacy remains, revered.
For every stone they shaped with care,
Holds a soul that lingers there.

33. A Night in the Forest

The forest hums with a quiet tune,
Beneath the stars and silver moon.
The leaves they rustle, the branches creak,
A symphony soft, a language unique.

The fireflies dance, their glow so bright,
A fleeting spark in the endless night.
The wolves they howl, the owls they call,
A melody born of the wild's thrall.

And in this song, the heart can rest,
A soul refreshed, a spirit blessed.
For nature's music, raw and free,
Is a hymn to life's eternity.

34. The Bridge of Mist

Across the valley, through the air,
A bridge of mist hangs light and fair.
Its arches gleam, its path unknown,
A passage spun of dreams alone.

The brave may tread its fragile span,
To lands unseen, to worlds unplanned.
Each step is soft, each breath is light,
A journey made through shadowed night.

But tread with care, for mist can fade,
And paths once clear may soon degrade.
Yet those who cross with hearts unbound,
Will find the dreams that life has crowned.

35. The Lonely Star

High above where silence dwells,
A single star its story tells.
It shines alone, its light so small,
Yet bold it burns, despite it all.

The darkness vast, the void so near,
Cannot snuff out its spark sincere.
For though alone, it still will blaze,
A beacon bright through endless haze.

Oh, lonely star, your heart is strong,
A testament to where we belong.
For every light, no matter how far,
Shines with purpose, as you are.

36. The Whispering Tide

The tide it whispers, soft and low,
A song it sings where waters flow.
It carries shells, it shapes the sand,
A sculptor's touch, a gentle hand.

Its voice is calm, yet strong and true,
A rhythm born of the ocean's blue.
And though it ebbs, and though it swells,
It keeps the secrets no one tells.

For in its waves, the world aligns,
A cosmic dance of endless signs.
The tide it whispers, soft and slow,
A song of life we'll always know.

37. The Watcher of the Sky

Upon the hills where shadows fall,
The watcher stands, so silent, tall.
Their eyes are fixed upon the night,
Where stars unfold their timeless light.

They count the heavens, they trace the line,
Of constellations bold, divine.
And though they stand in solitude,
Their heart is filled with gratitude.

For in the sky, a story gleams,
Of endless worlds and boundless dreams.
The watcher knows, though far they seem,
The stars are closer than we deem.

38. A Mirror of Dreams

A mirror stands in a quiet room,
Its surface smooth, its edges bloom.
And those who gaze will see within,

A reflection bright of what has been.

Yet deeper still, beyond the glass,
A world of dreams begins to amass.
A place unseen, a realm so vast,
Where futures blend with shadows cast.

Oh, mirror bright, what truths you hold,
A glimpse of courage, a tale untold.
For every dream you show so clear,
Is born of hope, not bound by fear.

39. The Silent Wind

The wind it moves with steps unseen,
Through fields of gold, through hills of green.
It whispers soft, it roars aloud,
A restless force, both fierce and proud.

It bends the trees, it shapes the land,
A fleeting touch, a guiding hand.
And though it wanders, never still,
It follows paths of ancient will.

For in its breath, a power lies,
To lift the earth, to kiss the skies.
The silent wind, so wild, so free,
A song of life's eternity.

40. The Flamekeeper

In shadowed halls, the flamekeeper stays,
Tending the fire that lights the days.
Their hands are steady, their watch is long,
Their heart is bold, their will is strong.

The fire burns with a golden hue,
A symbol bright, both old and new.
It warms the lost, it guides the blind,

A beacon true for all mankind.

And though the keeper fades with time,
Their flame endures, their duty prime.
For every spark they fed with care,
Will light the path for those who dare.

41. The River of Time

The river flows, both swift and slow,
A silent march where moments go.
Its waters clear, its depths unknown,
A path unmarked, a course unshown.

Through canyon walls and meadows wide,
It carries dreams on every tide.
Its voice a whisper, its song a sigh,
A fleeting tune beneath the sky.

Oh, river vast, you never pause,
You shape the world with unseen laws.
And those who drift within your stream,
Will find their lives a fleeting dream.

42. The Lost Ship

Upon the waves, a ghostly hull,
Its sails in shreds, its colors dull.
It drifts alone, no crew, no sound,
A spectral ship where none are found.

The winds they howl, the waves they rise,
Yet still it glides beneath dark skies.
Its course unknown, its tale untold,
A vessel lost in ocean's hold.

And those who glimpse its haunting form,
Will feel a chill both deep and warm.

For every ship, though lost at sea,
Holds dreams of what can never be.

43. The Silent Choir

In the chapel where no words are said,
The silent choir lifts the dead.
Their voices rise without a sound,
A melody that knows no bounds.

The candles flicker, the shadows dance,
A hymn of peace, a solemn trance.
Each note unseen, each tone unspoken,
A bridge of hope where hearts are broken.

Oh, silent choir, your song is clear,
A solace found for all who hear.
For even in the deepest pain,
Your quiet tune will still remain.

44. The Eternal Flame

Within the cave where darkness lies,
A single flame reflects the skies.
Its glow is steady, its warmth is pure,
A light eternal, strong and sure.

It knows no fear, it fears no wind,
Its fire lives where all rescind.
And those who find its sacred glow,
Will feel a peace they'll always know.

Oh, flame so bright, though small you seem,
You light the path of every dream.
For in your glow, the world will see,
A spark of hope, a destiny.

45. The Guardian Oak

Beneath its boughs, the earth stands still,
A silent guard upon the hill.
Its branches wide, its roots so deep,
A timeless giant where shadows sleep.

The seasons turn, the winds will howl,
Yet still it stands through storm and foul.
Its bark is scarred, its leaves may fall,
But in its heart, it holds it all.

Oh, guardian oak, your strength inspires,
A beacon bold through life's harsh fires.
For though the world may shift and sway,
Your roots remain, a steadfast stay.

46. The Song of the Horizon

The horizon calls, its voice so clear,
A promise bold to those who hear.
Its line is endless, its path untamed,
A place where dreams are unashamed.

The sky it bends, the sun will rise,
A meeting place of earth and skies.
And those who chase its fleeting glow,
Will find the truths they long to know.

Oh, horizon wide, your song is sweet,
A melody where dreams can meet.
For every heart that dares to stray,
Will find its home along your way.

47. The Winter King

The Winter King upon his throne,
His crown of frost, his heart of stone.
He rules the lands of ice and snow,
A kingdom vast where cold winds blow.

His breath is chill, his touch is freeze,
He whispers through the barren trees.
Yet in his reign, a beauty lies,
A frozen world beneath the skies.

Oh, Winter King, though harsh you seem,
You guard the earth in quiet dream.
For in your frost, the seeds will sleep,
And life shall wake when spring does creep.

48. The Whispering Brook

The brook it murmurs, soft and clear,
A soothing voice to all who hear.
Its waters dance through mossy stones,
A melody that soothes the bones.

It knows the song of forest deep,
Where shadows play and secrets sleep.
Its gentle flow will carve the earth,
A quiet hymn of life and birth.

Oh, whispering brook, your tune is kind,
A solace sweet for heart and mind.
For in your flow, the soul will find,
A peace that's pure, a love unlined.

49. The Lantern's Glow

Through darkest nights, the lantern burns,
A guiding light for all who yearn.
Its golden flame, a steady friend,
A beacon bright where shadows end.

The winds may blow, the storms may rage,
Yet still it shines through every stage.
Its glow a promise, soft yet clear,
A comfort found for all who near.

Oh, lantern bright, your warmth inspires,
A flame that lives through life's desires.
For even in the deepest gloom,
Your light will shine, your hope will bloom.

50. The Ocean's Mirror

The ocean gleams like polished glass,
A mirror vast where clouds will pass.
Its surface calm, its depths unknown,
A world of wonders all its own.

The sky it holds within its face,
A boundless blue, a timeless space.
And those who gaze upon its glow,
Will feel the peace that waters know.

Oh, ocean bright, your beauty sings,
A melody of boundless things.
For in your depths, the soul can see,
A mirror vast of eternity.

51. The Fire Within

A fire burns within the soul,
A restless flame that seeks its goal.
Its embers glow, its heat consumes,
A passion fierce, a light that looms.

It cannot die, it will not fade,
Through trials vast and plans mislaid.
For in its heart, a purpose clear,
A call to rise, a voice to hear.

Oh, fire within, your strength is true,
A spark that guides, a force anew.
For every soul that fans your flame,
Will find the path to love and name.

52. The Shadow's Edge

The shadow falls upon the land,
A fleeting mark of time's own hand.
Its edge is soft, its reach is wide,
A border drawn 'tween light and tide.

It dances bold, it hides, it sways,
A phantom born of light's own gaze.
And though it fades when night takes hold,
It leaves its mark in stories told.

Oh, shadow soft, your grace is clear,
A fleeting friend that lingers near.
For in your dance, the world will see,
A truth that lies in mystery.

53. The Calling Wind

The wind it calls, its voice so free,
A whisper bold from sky to sea.
It carries tales, it spreads the sound,
Of worlds unseen, of dreams unbound.

Its touch is soft, its power vast,
A force that shapes, a song that lasts.
And those who hear its quiet tone,
Will find their hearts no longer alone.

Oh, calling wind, your voice inspires,
A hymn that wakes the soul's desires.
For in your breath, the world will know,
The endless paths where dreams can go.

54. The Endless Stair

A stair it climbs, through earth and sky,
Its steps unnumbered, its purpose high.
It winds through clouds, it bends through stone,

A path to realms both vast and unknown.

Each step is hard, each rise is steep,
A climb that tests the heart's own deep.
Yet those who dare its height to face,
Will find a world of boundless grace.

Oh, endless stair, your call is clear,
A journey grand for those who hear.
For in your climb, the soul will find,
A peace that lives beyond the mind.

55. The Realm of Dreams

Beyond the veil where shadows drift,
A realm awaits, a timeless gift.
Its fields are gold, its rivers bright,
A boundless world of endless night.

The dreamers walk with hearts so free,
Through star-kissed skies and crystal seas.
Their fears dissolve, their hopes take flight,
In this domain of pure delight.

But dreams are fleeting, a fragile glow,
A fleeting path where few may go.
Yet in their light, the soul can find,
A fleeting peace for heart and mind.

56. The Keeper of the Tide

Upon the shore where waters break,
A keeper stands for ocean's sake.
Their eyes like storms, their heart like waves,
A soul that guards the ocean's graves.

The tide it bows beneath their hand,

A force they guide, a life they command.
And though they watch with solemn care,
The keeper longs for skies elsewhere.

Yet still they stand, their duty clear,
A guardian bold of waters near.
For in the tides, their purpose lies,
A bond that stretches to the skies.

57. The Valley of Echoes

In the valley where echoes play,
The past and present blend each day.
The mountains hum, the rivers sing,
A symphony of everything.

Each voice is clear, yet none is whole,
A fragment sung from every soul.
And those who walk this sacred land,
Will hear the songs of life firsthand.

Oh, valley bright, your music calls,
A hymn that echoes through your halls.
For in your voice, the world can hear,
A harmony both vast and near.

58. The Painter of Skies

The painter works with brush in hand,
Creating worlds both bold and grand.
Their canvas vast, their palette wide,
The endless stretch of heaven's tide.

With strokes of gold, they draw the dawn,
With hues of pink, the night is gone.
And when the sun begins to fade,
They blend the stars, a soft cascade.

Oh, painter bold, your art inspires,

A vision bright, a heart's desires.
For in your skies, the soul will find,
A beauty pure, a peace refined.

59. The Shepherd's Vigil

The shepherd stands beneath the moon,
Their watchful eyes a solemn tune.
The flock it grazes, the wolves they wait,
A fragile dance of love and fate.

The stars they shine, the fields are wide,
The shepherd walks where shadows hide.
Their steps are soft, their heart is kind,
A soul that guards, a peace defined.

Oh, shepherd brave, your path is true,
A life of care, a heart so blue.
For in your vigil, the world can see,
A quiet strength, a harmony.

60. The Dance of Flames

The fire dances, bold and bright,
A fleeting glow in endless night.
Its embers rise, its sparks take flight,
A living song of warmth and light.

It crackles soft, it roars aloud,
A force untamed, both fierce and proud.
Yet in its heart, a peace resides,
A power pure that time abides.

Oh, dancing flame, your rhythm sings,
A melody of countless things.
For in your glow, the heart can see,
A fleeting glimpse of eternity.

61. The Road of Stone

A road it winds through hill and vale,
A path of stone, a timeless trail.
Its surface worn by countless feet,
A journey grand, a tale complete.

The travelers walk with dreams in hand,
Through golden fields, through shifting sand.
Each step they take, each mile they roam,
Brings them closer to their home.

Oh, road of stone, your call is clear,
A path that spans both far and near.
For every step upon your way,
Is part of life's eternal play.

62. The Bell of Twilight

The bell it tolls as twilight falls,
A solemn sound through ancient halls.
Its echo rolls through dusk and haze,
A quiet hymn to end the days.

The stars awake, the moon takes flight,
And darkness claims the fading light.
Yet in its tone, a peace is found,
A gentle calm, a soothing sound.

Oh, bell of dusk, your chime is sweet,
A melody where night and day meet.
For in your song, the world can find,
A fleeting joy, a peace of mind.

63. The Whispering Leaves

The leaves they whisper in the breeze,
A gentle tune through ancient trees.
Their voices soft, their words unclear,
Yet still they sing for all to hear.

The forest hums with life unseen,
A world of gold, a realm of green.
And those who walk beneath its shade,
Will feel the peace the leaves have made.

Oh, whispering leaves, your song is true,
A melody of earth and dew.
For in your tune, the heart will find,
A solace sweet, a love unlined.

64. The Forgotten Gate

A gate it stands in a shadowed glen,
A portal lost to the world of men.
Its iron worn, its hinges weak,
A doorway old, a path unique.

Beyond its frame, the woods grow wild,
A realm untouched, a nature's child.
And those who step through rusted arch,
Will find a world where wonders march.

Oh, gate so lost, your secret keep,
A passage grand where dreams can leap.
For in your arms, the soul can stray,
To lands beyond the light of day.

65. The Solitary Flame

In the lantern by the sea,
A flame burns bright for all to see.
Its golden glow, a steady friend,
A beacon bold where darkness ends.

The storms may rage, the winds may cry,
But still it burns beneath the sky.
A light of hope, a flame of grace,
A guide for all who seek its face.

Oh, solitary flame, your warmth inspires,
A spark that lives through life's desires.
For in your glow, the soul will see,
A path of peace, a destiny.

66. The Watchtower's Gaze

Upon the cliffs where waves do crash,
A watchtower stands, its shadows cast.
Its walls of stone, its steps so steep,
A guardian bold where oceans leap.

The keeper walks with steady care,
Their eyes on seas both wide and fair.
And though the storms may hide the skies,
Their vigil lasts, their courage flies.

Oh, watchtower tall, your strength is true,
A symbol proud of skies so blue.
For in your gaze, the world will see,
A steadfast love for eternity.

67. The Rainmaker

The rainmaker lifts their hands to the sky,
A plea for life where the earth runs dry.
Their dance is bold, their spirit free,
A harmony with eternity.

The clouds they form, the winds they rise,
A storm is born beneath their cries.
And when the rain begins to fall,
It quenches life, it touches all.

Oh, rainmaker bold, your gift is clear,
A love that flows both far and near.
For in your storm, the world can see,
A promise born of destiny.

68. The Sky's Embrace

The sky wraps earth in endless blue,
A tender touch both old and new.
Its clouds drift soft, its winds caress,
A silent hymn of boundlessness.

It holds the sun in warm embrace,
It shields the moon in soft-spun lace.
And though its storms may rage and cry,
Its love endures, it cannot die.

Oh, sky so vast, your grace is clear,
A guardian bold, forever near.
For in your arms, the world does rest,
A cradle pure, a heart expressed.

69. The Forgotten Throne

In a hall where silence reigns,
A throne remains though none remains.
Its gold is worn, its jewels are dim,
A relic left in shadows grim.

The king who sat is dust and lore,
A name now lost forevermore.
Yet still the throne, with quiet pride,
Remembers all who lived and died.

Oh, throne so grand, your tale is vast,
A monument to ages past.
For in your seat, the echoes ring,
Of fleeting crowns and mortal kings.

70. The Starry Path

The stars align to mark a way,
A path unseen by light of day.

Its stones are dreams, its guide the night,
A road of wonder, pure delight.

Each step is soft, each turn unknown,
A journey far from flesh and bone.
And those who walk its starlit trail,
Will find a truth that will prevail.

Oh, starry path, your glow is kind,
A guide for those who seek to find.
For in your light, the soul will soar,
To realms unseen forevermore.

71. The Lighthouse Keeper's Song

Upon the cliffs where waves do pound,
The keeper hums a mournful sound.
Their lamp it burns through darkest night,
A beacon clear, a guiding light.

The storms may rise, the winds may wail,
Yet still they stand, their duty pale.
And though their heart is worn with years,
Their flame endures, it calms their fears.

Oh, keeper bold, your vigil stays,
A silent hymn through endless days.
For in your light, the world can see,
A love that guards eternity.

72. The Forest Cathedral

The forest stands in sacred glow,
Its arches high, its shadows low.
A cathedral vast, a holy hall,
Where whispers rise and spirits call.

Its pillars wide, its roof the skies,
A temple built where silence lies.

And those who tread its hallowed floor,
Will find a peace unseen before.

Oh, forest bright, your grace is true,
A realm of green, a world of blue.
For in your shade, the heart will know,
A sanctuary where life will grow.

73. The Desert's Voice

The desert speaks in tones so low,
A quiet hymn where few will go.
Its sands they shift, its dunes they sigh,
A world of gold beneath the sky.

The winds they carve, the sun does blaze,
A timeless dance through endless days.
And though its touch is harsh and bare,
A beauty raw lingers there.

Oh, desert vast, your voice is clear,
A song of life both far and near.
For in your heart, the soul can see,
A strength that blooms eternally.

74. The Tower in the Mist

The tower stands where mists do cling,
A spire lost where echoes sing.
Its stones are cold, its halls are bare,
A lonely watch in the dampened air.

The world forgets its ancient form,
Its purpose lost to time's great storm.
Yet still it stands, a ghostly mark,
A memory bright within the dark.

Oh, tower tall, your strength remains,
A monument to life's refrains.

For in your walls, the past will stay,
A whisper bold of yesterday.

75. The Bridge Beneath the Moon

Beneath the moon, the bridge does glow,
A quiet arch where waters flow.
Its stones are worn, its surface fine,
A passage built through love and time.

The travelers tread with hearts so light,
Across its span in silvered night.
And though its strength may fade with years,
Its soul remains, it calms their fears.

Oh, bridge so bright, your path inspires,
A journey bold through life's desires.
For in your span, the world can find,
A bond that ties both heart and mind.

76. The Song of the Meadowlark

The meadowlark sings at break of day,
A melody where dreams do play.
Its voice is clear, its tune is bright,
A golden thread in morning light.

The grasses sway, the flowers bloom,
Each note a gift, each sound a plume.
And those who hear its simple song,
Will find their hearts where they belong.

Oh, meadowlark, your voice is true,
A hymn of earth, a sky of blue.
For in your tune, the world will see,
A joy that flows eternally.

77. The Spirit of the Mountain

The mountain breathes, its heart so wide,
A spirit bold that cannot hide.
Its peaks are high, its valleys deep,
A world of stone where whispers sleep.

Its voice is low, its soul is vast,
A guardian strong of ages past.
And those who climb its towering form,
Will find a strength to weather storms.

Oh, mountain grand, your call is clear,
A challenge bold, a force sincere.
For in your heights, the soul will find,
A courage fierce, a peace refined.

78. The Harbor's Peace

The harbor sleeps as waves do roll,
A quiet home for every soul.
Its waters calm, its docks so still,
A sanctuary where hearts can heal.

The ships they rest, their sails unwound,
Their journeys paused on sacred ground.
And though the sea may call once more,
The harbor waits, its arms assure.

Oh, harbor kind, your peace is true,
A shelter bold beneath the blue.
For in your calm, the world can see,
A refuge found eternally.

79. The Traveler's Rest

The traveler stops where paths converge,
A haven found at twilight's urge.
Their pack is worn, their steps are slow,
A quiet peace begins to grow.

The hearth it warms, the bread it feeds,
A comfort born of simple needs.
And though their journey still remains,
The rest they find will soothe their pains.

Oh, traveler's rest, your gift is clear,
A place of calm for hearts held near.
For in your walls, the weary see,
A fleeting taste of eternity.

80. The Candle's Last Glow

The candle burns its final flame,
A fleeting spark that knows no shame.
Its wax it melts, its wick grows thin,
A gentle end, a soft within.

Its light it fades, yet still it glows,
A quiet love the darkness knows.
And though it dies, it leaves behind,
A warmth that lingers in the mind.

Oh, candle bright, your flame inspires,
A final spark, a soul's desires.
For even in your last embrace,
You light the world with tender grace.

101. The Wind's Secrets

The wind it whispers soft and low,
A tale of places few will go.
It carries scents of lands afar,
Of oceans deep and evening stars.

Its voice is light, its call is clear,
A fleeting sound that lingers near.
And though it travels far and wide,

Its secrets stay where hearts confide.

Oh, restless wind, your path is free,
A journey vast through sky and sea.
For in your breath, the world can hear,
A timeless song both far and near.

102. The Watcher's Silence

The watcher stands on the cliffs alone,
A shadow cast in twilight's tone.
Their gaze is fixed on the horizon wide,
Where sun meets sea and secrets hide.

They do not speak, they make no sound,
Their feet are firm on sacred ground.
And though the years may come and go,
The watcher guards what none may know.

Oh, silent soul, your vigil stays,
Through endless nights and fleeting days.
For in your stillness, the world can see,
A quiet strength, a mystery.

103. The Lantern in the Fog

Through foggy streets where shadows creep,
A lantern glows where secrets sleep.
Its light is faint, its flame is small,
Yet still it guides through it all.

The mist it wraps the world in gray,
A shroud that hides both night and day.
Yet in its glow, a path appears,
A beacon bright through doubts and fears.

Oh, lantern soft, your light is clear,
A fragile flame that draws us near.
For in your glow, the heart will find,

A courage rare, a peace refined.

104. The Pilgrim's Prayer

The pilgrim walks with steady pace,
Through winding paths, through open space.
Their feet are tired, their heart is worn,
Yet still they seek where dreams are born.

Each step they take, a quiet plea,
To find the truth they long to see.
And though the road is harsh and long,
Their spirit hums a quiet song.

Oh, pilgrim bold, your journey's true,
A path of hope through skies of blue.
For in your prayer, the world can hear,
A love that spans both far and near.

105. The Mirror of the Moon

Beneath the moon where waters gleam,
A mirror lies to catch its beam.
Its surface smooth, its light so clear,
A fleeting glimpse of worlds so near.

The stars they dance upon its face,
A quiet hymn, a boundless grace.
And those who gaze into its glow,
Will feel the truths the waters show.

Oh, mirror bright, your light inspires,
A path to dreams, a heart's desires.
For in your glow, the soul can see,
A beauty born of mystery.

106. The Weaver's Loom

The weaver works with hands so kind,

A thread of dreams through time entwined.
Their loom is vast, their vision wide,
A tapestry where lives collide.

Each thread they spin, a story told,
Of love and loss, of hearts so bold.
And though their work may never end,
Each stitch is made with love to mend.

Oh, weaver wise, your art is true,
A life of care, a heart of blue.
For in your craft, the world can see,
A bond that ties eternity.

107. The Sea's Cradle

The sea it rocks with gentle care,
A cradle vast, a love so rare.
Its waves they sing, its tides they sigh,
A soothing hymn beneath the sky.

The ships they drift, the stars they gleam,
A quiet world where dreamers dream.
And though its depths are dark and wide,
Its surface holds a mother's pride.

Oh, sea so grand, your heart is kind,
A solace found for heart and mind.
For in your waves, the soul can see,
A cradle bright of eternity.

108. The Flame's Whisper

The candle flickers in the dark,
Its flame a tiny, fleeting spark.
It whispers soft, it hums so low,
A song of warmth where shadows grow.

Its light may waver, yet still it stays,

A golden thread through night's long maze.
And though its life is short and sweet,
Its warmth remains, a soft heartbeat.

Oh, whispering flame, your glow inspires,
A quiet hymn of heart's desires.
For in your light, the world can see,
A hope that burns eternally.

109. The Mountain's Echo

The mountain speaks in tones so grand,
A voice that rolls through all the land.
Its echoes rise, its whispers fall,
A hymn that binds the world to all.

The rocks they hum, the rivers sing,
A melody of everything.
And those who climb its towering face,
Will hear the songs of boundless grace.

Oh, mountain bold, your voice is true,
A symphony of earth and blue.
For in your echoes, the heart will find,
A harmony of soul and mind.

110. The Frozen Lake

Beneath the frost, the water sleeps,
A silent world where stillness keeps.
Its surface shines like polished glass,
A mirror bright where footsteps pass.

The trees they guard its icy form,
A crystal plain through winter's storm.
And though it rests in frozen peace,
Its heart still beats, it will not cease.

Oh, frozen lake, your calm is clear,

A quiet strength for all who near.
For in your stillness, the world can see,
A beauty born of serenity.

111. The Midnight Bell

The bell it tolls at midnight's hour,
A solemn sound of fleeting power.
Its chime is deep, its tone so pure,
A call to hearts both strong and sure.

The stars they listen, the moon does glow,
A quiet world where time runs slow.
And those who hear its gentle ring,
Will find the peace its notes can bring.

Oh, midnight bell, your sound inspires,
A fleeting calm, a soul's desires.
For in your chime, the world can see,
A harmony of unity.

112. The Meadow's Glow

The meadow hums with quiet light,
A golden field in fading night.
Its flowers bloom, its grasses sway,
A gentle song at break of day.

The bees they hum, the breeze it sighs,
A lullaby beneath the skies.
And those who walk its soft embrace,
Will feel the warmth of nature's grace.

Oh, meadow bright, your glow is clear,
A haven sweet for hearts held near.
For in your light, the soul can find,
A joy that lingers, undefined.

113. The River's Lament

The river sighs as it winds its way,
Through valleys wide and skies of gray.
Its waters clear, its heart so deep,
A place where dreams and memories sleep.

It carries tales of mountain peaks,
Of forests green and ocean creeks.
Yet in its flow, a sadness grows,
A longing for where no one knows.

Oh, river vast, your voice is low,
A mournful tune where time does flow.
For in your depths, the world can see,
A reflection vast of eternity.

114. The Star-Seeker

The seeker climbs the hills at night,
Their eyes alight with starlit sight.
They trace the paths where comets glide,
Through endless skies, where dreams reside.

Their heart is bold, their will is free,
They long to touch eternity.
And though the stars remain so far,
Their soul becomes a burning star.

Oh, seeker bright, your quest inspires,
A soul ignited with fierce desires.
For in your gaze, the world will see,
A yearning boundless as the sea.

115. The Winter Song

The snow it falls in a hushed refrain,
A melody soft, a quiet gain.

Its touch is cold, yet oddly warm,
A fleeting grace in winter's storm.

The trees stand still, their branches bare,
Their whispers lost in frosty air.
Yet in the stillness, a song takes flight,
A hymn to honor the endless night.

Oh, winter's song, your notes are clear,
A gentle call for hearts to hear.
For in your silence, life will find,
A harmony of heart and mind.

116. The Flame and the Shadow

The flame it dances, bold and bright,
A flickering spark in the heart of night.
Its shadow sways upon the wall,
A silent partner to its call.

The fire burns with a life of its own,
Its warmth a gift, its spirit unknown.
Yet in its glow, the shadow stays,
A quiet echo through its blaze.

Oh, flame so bright, your truth is clear,
A dual force both far and near.
For in your light, the world can see,
A balance born of harmony.

117. The Forgotten Chapel

Deep in the woods, where sunlight fades,
A chapel stands in twilight's shades.
Its walls are cracked, its steeple worn,
A place where prayers were once reborn.

The candles flicker, though none attend,
A sacred light that will not bend.

And though its halls are filled with dust,
Its spirit lingers, strong and just.

Oh, chapel lost, your heart remains,
A quiet strength through life's refrains.
For in your peace, the world can find,
A solace pure, a love refined.

118. The Whispering Sands

The desert sings in whispers low,
A voice that shifts where winds do blow.
Its grains they dance, its dunes they rise,
A living hymn beneath the skies.

Its silence speaks of endless days,
Of scorching suns and twilight's haze.
And those who walk its boundless plain,
Will find its truths in joy and pain.

Oh, desert vast, your voice inspires,
A quiet strength through harsh desires.
For in your sands, the soul can see,
A path to grace, a destiny.

119. The Song of the Wolves

The wolves they howl in the forest deep,
A haunting call where shadows creep.
Their voices rise, their tones align,
A melody fierce, a tune divine.

The moon it listens, the stars reply,
A quiet bond between earth and sky.
And though their song is wild and free,
It carries a truth for all to see.

Oh, wolves so bold, your hymn is clear,
A call of life both far and near.

For in your cry, the world will know,
A love that lingers, a strength to grow.

120. The Tides of Change

The tides they turn with a steady hand,
A force that shapes both sea and land.
Their ebb and flow, their rise and fall,
A rhythm vast that binds us all.

The waters pull, the shores they yield,
A dance eternal, a bond revealed.
And though the waves may crash and break,
Their purpose clear, their truth awake.

Oh, tides so vast, your song inspires,
A hymn that soothes, a heart's desires.
For in your flow, the world can find,
A strength eternal, a peace aligned.

121. The Candle in the Window

The candle glows with a golden light,
A beacon bold in the heart of night.
Its flame it flickers, yet still it stays,
A quiet guide through endless days.

The house it guards, its hearth so warm,
A refuge safe from life's great storm.
And those who see its gentle gleam,
Will find their hearts in restful dream.

Oh, candle bright, your light is clear,
A fragile flame that draws us near.
For in your glow, the soul can see,
A love that burns eternally.

122. The Traveler's Song

The traveler hums as they tread the road,
A melody born of life's great load.
Their pack is light, their steps are sure,
Their heart is free, their soul is pure.

The fields they pass, the skies they meet,
Each moment bright, each step so sweet.
And though the journey has no end,
The path itself becomes their friend.

Oh, traveler bold, your song is true,
A hymn of life through skies so blue.
For in your voice, the world can hear,
A boundless joy both far and near.

123. The Forest of Shadows

The forest hums with a quiet breath,
A place of life, a hint of death.
Its shadows dance, its trees they sigh,
A realm of wonder beneath the sky.

The leaves they fall, the roots they grow,
A cycle vast where spirits flow.
And those who tread its sacred floor,
Will find a peace unseen before.

Oh, forest deep, your voice is kind,
A hymn of earth, a heart aligned.
For in your shade, the world can see,
A beauty born of mystery.

124. The Broken Clock

The clock it ticks, though hands are still,
A quiet beat, a tempered will.
Its face is worn, its chime is low,
A relic lost to time's own flow.

And yet it stands, its purpose clear,
A silent mark of every year.
For though it fades, its heart remains,
A symbol true of life's refrains.

Oh, broken clock, your tale inspires,

125. The Lighthouse of Dreams

Upon the shore, where waters gleam,
A lighthouse stands, a beacon of dreams.
Its light it turns, its glow it casts,
A guide for those adrift and vast.

The waves they crash, the winds they cry,
But still it shines beneath the sky.
And though the storms may shake the land,
Its tower stands, a steady hand.

Oh, lighthouse bold, your heart is true,
A light of hope through skies of blue.
For in your glow, the world can see,
A path to love, a destiny.

126. The Snowflake's Journey

A snowflake drifts through winter's air,
A fragile form beyond compare.
Its crystals shine, its pattern rare,
A fleeting beauty none can spare.

It lands so soft upon the earth,
A silent witness to its birth.
And though it melts in time's embrace,
Its fleeting life holds endless grace.

Oh, snowflake bright, your tale is clear,

A moment pure, a truth sincere.
For in your fall, the world can see,
A glimpse of life's fragility.

127. The Song of the Horizon

The horizon hums with a quiet tone,
A melody vast, a tune unknown.
Its line it bends, its skies unfold,
A canvas wide of blue and gold.

It calls to hearts that long to stray,
To wander paths where dreams convey.
And though its edge may seem so far,
Its song is clear, a guiding star.

Oh, horizon wide, your voice inspires,
A boundless hope, a soul's desires.
For in your call, the heart will find,
A journey bold through space and time.

128. The Forest Sentinel

Deep in the woods where shadows dwell,
A sentinel stands, a sacred spell.
Its branches stretch, its roots dig deep,
A guardian bold where spirits sleep.

The seasons turn, the winds may howl,
But still it stands through sun and foul.
Its bark is scarred, its leaves may fall,
Yet in its heart, it holds it all.

Oh, sentinel wise, your strength inspires,
A symbol grand through life's desires.
For in your shade, the soul can see,
A timeless bond with eternity.

129. The Quiet Stream

The stream it flows with a gentle tune,
A liquid path beneath the moon.
Its waters clear, its ripples small,
A soothing voice that touches all.

It carries whispers of mountain springs,
Of distant skies and eagle wings.
And those who rest beside its flow,
Will feel the peace its currents show.

Oh, quiet stream, your song is kind,
A melody for heart and mind.
For in your flow, the world can hear,
A harmony both far and near.

130. The Candle's Vigil

The candle burns through endless night,
A fragile flame, a steady light.
Its wax it melts, its wick grows thin,
Yet still it guards the dark within.

The shadows bend, the winds they sigh,
But still it shines, it will not die.
A faithful flame through trials vast,
A quiet glow that will outlast.

Oh, candle bright, your light inspires,
A beacon true through life's desires.
For in your flame, the soul can see,
A strength that burns eternally.

131. The Song of the Stars

The stars they sing in the velvet sky,
A melody vast, a lullaby.
Their voices soft, their notes so clear,
A hymn of love for all to hear.

They whisper tales of worlds afar,
Of endless dreams and fallen stars.
And though their light may seem so small,
Their song unites and touches all.

Oh, stars so bright, your tune inspires,
A harmony through life's desires.
For in your song, the heart will find,
A beauty vast, a peace divine.

132. The Solitary Rose

Amidst the weeds, the rose does bloom,
A fragile beauty in nature's room.
Its petals soft, its color bold,
A treasure rare in a world so cold.

The thorns it bears, a shield so tight,
A quiet strength in morning light.
And though it stands alone, unseen,
Its heart remains forever green.

Oh, rose so bright, your grace inspires,
A testament to life's desires.
For in your bloom, the world can see,
A beauty pure, a destiny.

133. The Eternal Flame

Within the hearth where shadows fall,
The flame it burns, it lights it all.
Its warmth it gives, its glow it shares,
A tender love that always cares.

The winters pass, the nights grow long,
Yet still it hums its quiet song.
And those who gather near its light,
Will find a peace through

134. The Keeper of Shadows

In twilight halls where silence grows,
The keeper walks where no one knows.
Their cloak is dark, their steps are light,
A guardian born of endless night.

They gather fears, they soothe the mind,
They shield the dreams that fear confined.
And though unseen, their watch remains,
A silent force through life's refrains.

Oh, keeper bold, your path inspires,
A steady hand through life's desires.
For in your care, the heart will find,
A solace deep, a peace unlined.

135. The Sky's Cathedral

The clouds they drift in endless white,
A cathedral vast in morning light.
Its arches bend, its windows glow,
A masterpiece where breezes flow.

The sun it sings, the winds reply,
A hymn of love through endless sky.
And those who gaze upon its height,
Will feel the grace of boundless flight.

Oh, sky so wide, your beauty reigns,
A sanctuary free of chains.
For in your space, the soul can see,
A temple built for eternity.

136. The Silent Grove

Beneath the trees where shadows rest,
The grove it hums, its heart expressed.
Its leaves they murmur, its branches sway,
A quiet song through night and day.

The earth is soft, the air is still,
A sacred calm, a timeless will.
And those who walk its shaded floor,
Will find a peace they knew before.

Oh, grove so deep, your song inspires,
A refuge bold for life's desires.
For in your calm, the heart will see,
A harmony with eternity.

137. The Sailor's Star

The sailor stands beneath the sky,
A restless soul with wondering eye.
Their compass lost, their map unclear,
Yet still they sail where stars appear.

The north star shines, its glow so bright,
A beacon bold through endless night.
And though the waves may rise and fall,
Its guiding light will lead through all.

Oh, sailor bold, your heart inspires,
A journey vast through fierce desires.
For in your star, the world can see,
A path of hope through stormy seas.

138. The Clockmaker's Tune

The clockmaker hums a steady tone,
A melody soft, a tune their own.
Their hands they move with tender care,
Through ticking worlds both bright and rare.

Each gear they turn, each spring they wind,
A quiet dance of heart and mind.
And though their art is slow and small,
Its rhythm binds the lives of all.

Oh, clockmaker, your work inspires,
A symphony through time's desires.
For in your hands, the world will find,
A harmony of clock and mind.

139. The Shoreline's Edge

The shore it stands where worlds collide,
A meeting place for sea and tide.
Its sands they shift, its waves they dance,
A fleeting grace, a bold romance.

The shells they glimmer, the breeze it sighs,
A symphony beneath the skies.
And those who walk its endless span,
Will find the truths of sea and land.

Oh, shoreline wide, your beauty sings,
A melody of boundless things.
For in your reach, the heart can see,
A love that spans eternity.

140. The Nightingale's Song

The nightingale sings in shadows deep,
A voice that stirs where silence sleeps.
Its notes they rise, its tune takes flight,
A melody born of endless night.

The moon it listens, the stars reply,
A harmony that graces the sky.
And those who hear its gentle sound,
Will find their hearts in beauty bound.

Oh, nightingale, your song inspires,
A hymn that lights the soul's desires.
For in your voice, the world will see,
A love that lasts eternally.

141. The Bridge of Time

The bridge it spans through years untold,
A pathway bright, a journey bold.
Its arches gleam with wisdom's glow,
A quiet path where dreamers go.

Each step it holds, each soul it bears,
A witness vast to life's affairs.
And though its stones may wear with age,
Its strength remains, a timeless stage.

Oh, bridge of time, your span inspires,
A crossing vast through life's desires.
For in your reach, the heart will see,
A bond that links eternity.

142. The Harp of Winds

The winds they pluck the harp of trees,
A melody soft, a song of seas.
Each note it plays, a whispered tone,
A hymn of life through wood and stone.

The grasses hum, the rivers sing,
A symphony of everything.
And those who pause to hear its song,
Will find their hearts where they belong.

Oh, harp of winds, your tune inspires,
A harmony through life's desires.
For in your strings, the world will see,
A melody of unity.

143. The Desert Bloom

Amidst the sands where sun does reign,
A flower blooms in harsh terrain.
Its petals bright, its stem so bold,
A miracle in dunes of gold.

The winds they howl, the days are long,
Yet still it grows, so pure, so strong.
A symbol born of life's resolve,
A quiet truth where hearts evolve.

Oh, desert bloom, your grace inspires,
A beauty found through life's desires.
For in your bloom, the world can see,
A love that thrives eternally.

144. The Keeper of Dawn

At break of day, the keeper stands,
Their eyes on skies, their heart in hands.
They watch the sun as it ascends,
A light of hope that never ends.

The clouds they part, the shadows fade,
A golden path through night conveyed.
And though the dawn is brief and shy,
It leaves its mark upon the sky.

Oh, keeper bold, your watch inspires,
A strength that lights the soul's desires.
For in your gaze, the heart can see,
A beauty born of eternity.

This set brings us deeper into the collection—let me know if you'd
like more to continue! □

145. The Ocean's Embrace

The ocean stretches far and wide,
A boundless force, a gentle tide.
Its waves they kiss the golden sands,
A love that's felt by distant lands.

Its voice is low, its song serene,
A melody of worlds unseen.
And those who stand upon its shore,
Will feel its pull forevermore.

Oh, ocean vast, your heart inspires,
A hymn of life, of deep desires.
For in your depths, the soul will find,
A timeless bond with humankind.

146. The Lantern of Hope

Through stormy nights and endless rain,
A lantern burns through grief and pain.
Its golden glow, a steadfast flame,
A quiet guide that calls your name.

The shadows bend, the winds may wail,
But still it stands, it will not fail.
And those who follow where it leads,
Will find the strength their spirit needs.

Oh, lantern bright, your light inspires,
A beacon strong through life's desires.
For in your glow, the world can see,
A path of hope through destiny.

147. The Forest's Song

The forest hums with ancient tones,
A melody of roots and stones.
Its trees they sway, its leaves they dance,
A timeless hymn of circumstance.

The streams they sing, the winds reply,
A harmony beneath the sky.
And those who walk its sacred halls,
Will hear the tune that nature calls.

Oh, forest deep, your song inspires,
A hymn of life, of grand desires.
For in your music, the heart can see,
A beauty born of eternity.

148. The Dreamer's Path

The dreamer walks where none have been,
Through starlit skies and worlds within.
Their steps are light, their gaze is wide,
A wanderer lost in the great divide.

The stars they guide, the winds they call,
A journey vast, a truth for all.
And though their path is steep and long,
They tread with hope, they hum their song.

Oh, dreamer bold, your quest inspires,
A life alight with fierce desires.
For in your dreams, the world can see,
A boundless love, a destiny.

149. The Forgotten Star

A star it glimmers faint and small,
A lonely light that touches all.
Its glow is soft, its voice is near,
A quiet call for those who hear.

It tells of worlds beyond our own,
Of mysteries vast, of seeds unknown.
And though its shine may fade with years,
Its legacy endures in tears.

Oh, star so lost, your light inspires,
A beacon bold through life's desires.
For in your glow, the heart will find,
A love that lingers, unconfined.

150. The Traveler's Flame

The traveler lights their flame at night,
A beacon bright, a guiding light.
Its glow it casts on paths unknown,
A quiet warmth where fears are sown.

The road is long, the winds are cold,
But still the flame, it burns so bold.
And though the night may stretch for miles,
Its golden glow renews their smiles.

Oh, traveler's flame, your light inspires,
A spark of hope through life's desires.
For in your fire, the world can see,
A strength that burns eternally.

151. The Meadow's Whisper

The meadow whispers soft and low,
A gentle breeze where flowers grow.
Its grasses sway, its blossoms sing,
A melody of everything.

The bees they hum, the sun it glows,
A quiet calm the meadow shows.
And those who rest upon its ground,
Will feel the peace that it has found.

Oh, meadow bright, your grace inspires,
A haven pure through life's desires.
For in your fields, the soul can find,
A harmony with heart and

Here's the next **20 long, lyrical poems** to further expand this beautiful collection. Each poem is thoughtfully crafted to inspire and resonate deeply. □

152. The River's Memory

The river flows with whispers sweet,
Its currents sing where past and present meet.
It winds through valleys, soft and clear,
A timeless voice for all to hear.

Its waters carry stories old,
Of mountain springs and sands of gold.
And though it bends and finds the sea,
It leaves behind its memory.

Oh, river vast, your tale inspires,
A hymn of life, of deep desires.
For in your flow, the world can see,
A bond with time and destiny.

153. The Night's Embrace

The night unfolds with velvet arms,
Its stillness calm, its darkness charms.
The stars they glimmer, faint yet true,
A thousand lights in skies of blue.

Its silence soothes, its whispers low,
A sacred peace the shadows know.
And those who rest beneath its skies,
Will find their fears begin to die.

Oh, night so vast, your grace inspires,
A cradle soft for life's desires.
For in your arms, the world can see,
A solace deep, a mystery.

154. The Keeper of Flame

The keeper tends the hearth so bright,
A golden fire through endless night.
Their hands are steady, their heart is bold,
A guardian true of warmth untold.

The wood it burns, the embers glow,
A steady light where shadows grow.
And though the winds may howl and cry,
The keeper's flame will never die.

Oh, keeper strong, your work inspires,
A steady glow through life's desires.
For in your fire, the world can find,
A love that burns with heart aligned.

155. The Echoing Hills

The hills they hum in twilight's haze,
A quiet tune of ancient days.
Their echoes drift through time and space,
A melody the winds embrace.

The grasses wave, the stones they sigh,
A harmony beneath the sky.
And those who climb their gentle crest,
Will find a peace within their breast.

Oh, hills so wide, your song inspires,
A hymn of earth, of heart's desires.
For in your echoes, the world can see,
A beauty born of memory.

156. The Star-Crowned Tree

A tree it stands upon the hill,
Its branches wide, its roots so still.
The stars they rest upon its crown,
A radiant glow as night comes down.

Its leaves they shimmer, soft with dew,
A beacon bright through skies of blue.
And those who rest beneath its shade,
Will find a peace that does not fade.

Oh, tree so grand, your grace inspires,
A steadfast love through life's desires.
For in your glow, the heart will find,
A bond with stars and humankind.

157. The Wind's Waltz

The wind it waltzes through the air,
A partner bold, a dancer rare.
It bends the trees, it stirs the seas,
A graceful tune through land and breeze.

Its steps are soft, its voice is clear,
A melody that all can hear.
And those who feel its fleeting touch,
Will find a joy within its clutch.

Oh, wind so free, your dance inspires,
A motion vast through life's desires.
For in your flow, the world can see,
A rhythm born of unity.

158. The Forgotten Meadow

Beyond the hills where few will tread,
A meadow blooms where dreams are fed.
Its flowers wild, its grasses high,

A hidden realm beneath the sky.

The birds they sing, the bees they hum,
A gentle world where hearts become.
And those who walk its fragrant field,
Will find a truth the earth revealed.

Oh, meadow lost, your beauty sings,
A quiet hymn of timeless things.
For in your bloom, the soul can see,
A place of peace, a sanctuary.

159. The Song of Frost

The frost it paints with tender hand,
A fleeting art upon the land.
Its crystals gleam in morning light,
A fleeting spark of winter's night.

The trees they wear its silver cloak,
A quiet grace the dawn invokes.
And those who gaze upon its art,
Will find its beauty warms the heart.

Oh, frost so pure, your work inspires,
A fleeting joy through life's desires.
For in your chill, the world can see,
A fragile love, a mystery.

160. The Eternal Shore

The shore it stretches, soft and wide,
A meeting place for sea and tide.
Its sands they gleam beneath the sun,
A sacred bond where worlds are one.

The waves they dance, the breeze it sings,
A melody of boundless things.
And those who walk its golden span,

Will find their hearts where dreams began.

Oh, shore so vast, your grace inspires,
A bridge of hope through life's desires.
For in your sands, the world can see,
A love that flows eternally.

161. The Spirit of the Flame

The flame it flickers, wild yet true,
A living force of golden hue.
Its heat it gives, its light it shares,
A tender heart that always cares.

The shadows fade beneath its glow,
A warmth that all the world will know.
And though its life may fade in time,
Its spirit lingers, bold, sublime.

Oh, spirit bright, your fire inspires,
A steadfast love through life's desires.
For in your glow, the soul can find,
A strength that burns with heart aligned.

162. The Solitary Willow

The willow bends by the quiet stream,
Its branches trail as if in dream.
Its leaves they sigh, its roots dig deep,
A guardian born of shadows steep.

The water hums, the breezes play,
Yet still the willow holds its sway.
And those who sit beneath its bough,
Will feel its peace, its sacred vow.

Oh, willow wise, your grace inspires,
A gentle love through life's desires.
For in your shade, the world can see,

A quiet bond with eternity.

kkkHere's the next **20 long, lyrical poems** to further expand this beautiful collection. Each poem is thoughtfully crafted to inspire and resonate deeply. ☐

152. The River's Memory

The river flows with whispers sweet,
Its currents sing where past and present meet.
It winds through valleys, soft and clear,
A timeless voice for all to hear.

Its waters carry stories old,
Of mountain springs and sands of gold.
And though it bends and finds the sea,
It leaves behind its memory.

Oh, river vast, your tale inspires,
A hymn of life, of deep desires.
For in your flow, the world can see,
A bond with time and destiny.

153. The Night's Embrace

The night unfolds with velvet arms,
Its stillness calm, its darkness charms.
The stars they glimmer, faint yet true,
A thousand lights in skies of blue.

Its silence soothes, its whispers low,
A sacred peace the shadows know.
And those who rest beneath its skies,
Will find their fears begin to die.

Oh, night so vast, your grace inspires,
A cradle soft for life's desires.
For in your arms, the world can see,
A solace deep, a mystery.

154. The Keeper of Flame

The keeper tends the hearth so bright,
A golden fire through endless night.
Their hands are steady, their heart is bold,
A guardian true of warmth untold.

The wood it burns, the embers glow,
A steady light where shadows grow.
And though the winds may howl and cry,
The keeper's flame will never die.

Oh, keeper strong, your work inspires,
A steady glow through life's desires.
For in your fire, the world can find,
A love that burns with heart aligned.

155. The Echoing Hills

The hills they hum in twilight's haze,
A quiet tune of ancient days.
Their echoes drift through time and space,
A melody the winds embrace.

The grasses wave, the stones they sigh,
A harmony beneath the sky.
And those who climb their gentle crest,
Will find a peace within their breast.

Oh, hills so wide, your song inspires,
A hymn of earth, of heart's desires.
For in your echoes, the world can see,
A beauty born of memory.

156. The Star-Crowned Tree

A tree it stands upon the hill,
Its branches wide, its roots so still.
The stars they rest upon its crown,

A radiant glow as night comes down.

Its leaves they shimmer, soft with dew,
A beacon bright through skies of blue.
And those who rest beneath its shade,
Will find a peace that does not fade.

Oh, tree so grand, your grace inspires,
A steadfast love through life's desires.
For in your glow, the heart will find,
A bond with stars and humankind.

157. The Wind's Waltz

The wind it waltzes through the air,
A partner bold, a dancer rare.
It bends the trees, it stirs the seas,
A graceful tune through land and breeze.

Its steps are soft, its voice is clear,
A melody that all can hear.
And those who feel its fleeting touch,
Will find a joy within its clutch.

Oh, wind so free, your dance inspires,
A motion vast through life's desires.
For in your flow, the world can see,
A rhythm born of unity.

158. The Forgotten Meadow

Beyond the hills where few will tread,
A meadow blooms where dreams are fed.
Its flowers wild, its grasses high,
A hidden realm beneath the sky.

The birds they sing, the bees they hum,
A gentle world where hearts become.
And those who walk its fragrant field,

Will find a truth the earth revealed.

Oh, meadow lost, your beauty sings,
A quiet hymn of timeless things.
For in your bloom, the soul can see,
A place of peace, a sanctuary.

159. The Song of Frost

The frost it paints with tender hand,
A fleeting art upon the land.
Its crystals gleam in morning light,
A fleeting spark of winter's night.

The trees they wear its silver cloak,
A quiet grace the dawn invokes.
And those who gaze upon its art,
Will find its beauty warms the heart.

Oh, frost so pure, your work inspires,
A fleeting joy through life's desires.
For in your chill, the world can see,
A fragile love, a mystery.

160. The Eternal Shore

The shore it stretches, soft and wide,
A meeting place for sea and tide.
Its sands they gleam beneath the sun,
A sacred bond where worlds are one.

The waves they dance, the breeze it sings,
A melody of boundless things.
And those who walk its golden span,
Will find their hearts where dreams began.

Oh, shore so vast, your grace inspires,
A bridge of hope through life's desires.
For in your sands, the world can see,

A love that flows eternally.

161. The Spirit of the Flame

The flame it flickers, wild yet true,
A living force of golden hue.
Its heat it gives, its light it shares,
A tender heart that always cares.

The shadows fade beneath its glow,
A warmth that all the world will know.
And though its life may fade in time,
Its spirit lingers, bold, sublime.

Oh, spirit bright, your fire inspires,
A steadfast love through life's desires.
For in your glow, the soul can find,
A strength that burns with heart aligned.

162. The Solitary Willow

The willow bends by the quiet stream,
Its branches trail as if in dream.
Its leaves they sigh, its roots dig deep,
A guardian born of shadows steep.

The water hums, the breezes play,
Yet still the willow holds its sway.
And those who sit beneath its bough,
Will feel its peace, its sacred vow.

Oh, willow wise, your grace inspires,
A gentle love through life's desires.
For in your shade, the world can see,
A quiet bond with eternity.

163. The Flame keeper's Oath

Through storm and wind, the keeper stands,
The flame alive within their hands.
Its light is small, yet fierce and bold,
A fire pure, a story told.

The shadows press, the cold winds cry,
Yet still it burns beneath the sky.
For in their heart, a vow remains,
To guard the flame through joy and pain.

Oh, keeper strong, your duty inspires,
A steadfast will through life's desires.
For in your care, the world will see,
A light that shines eternally.

164. The Forgotten Harbor

The harbor sleeps where dreams are moored,
Its waters calm, its peace assured.
The ships they rest, their sails are furled,
A quiet pause in a restless world.

The moonlight glows, the stars look down,
A haven found where tides have crowned.
And those who linger in its embrace,
Will find the calm of a timeless space.

Oh, harbor kind, your heart inspires,
A cradle soft for life's desires.
For in your stillness, the soul can find,
A love that lingers, unconfined.

165. The Winter's Breath

The winter breathes with icy grace,
A frost that touches every place.
Its winds they howl, its whispers low,

A song of cold where shadows grow.

The trees they stand, their branches bare,
A solemn sight in frigid air.
Yet in its chill, a beauty lies,
A fleeting truth beneath the skies.

Oh, winter vast, your voice inspires,
A quiet peace through life's desires.
For in your cold, the world can see,
A fragile love in purity.

166. The Wanderer's Lament

The wanderer walks with weary feet,
Through paths unknown, where roads don't meet.
Their heart is heavy, their soul is tired,
Yet still they press, by dreams inspired.

The stars they guide, the winds they call,
A beacon bright when shadows fall.
And though their journey may not end,
The road itself becomes their friend.

Oh, wanderer bold, your quest inspires,
A life of hope, of deep desires.
For in your steps, the world can find,
A love that lingers, unconfined.

167. The Forest's Secret

The forest holds a quiet lore,
A mystery within its core.
Its trees they whisper, its shadows play,
A sacred tale that fades with day.

The roots they weave a hidden past,
A story deep, a truth that lasts.
And those who pause to feel its grace,

Will find a world of endless space.

Oh, forest deep, your secret inspires,
A hidden world through life's desires.
For in your shade, the heart can see,
A truth that lives eternally.

168. The Star-Kissed Plains

The plains they stretch beneath the sky,
A boundless world where stars reside.
Their grasses wave, their flowers bloom,
A sea of gold in twilight's room.

The moon it shines, the winds they sing,
A melody of everything.
And those who walk this endless field,
Will find a peace the stars revealed.

Oh, plains so wide, your heart inspires,
A gentle hymn through life's desires.
For in your glow, the world can see,
A bond with stars and eternity.

169. The Lantern in the Storm

The storm it rages fierce and wild,
The winds they howl, the seas defiled.
Yet through the dark, a lantern glows,
A beacon bright where courage shows.

Its flame is small, its light is weak,
Yet still it burns through stormy peaks.
And those who follow where it leads,
Will find the strength their spirit needs.

Oh, lantern bold, your light inspires,
A steady glow through life's desires.
For in your flame, the world can see,

A path through fear to destiny.

170. The Song of the Wolves

The wolves they sing beneath the moon,
A haunting hymn, a timeless tune.
Their voices rise in echoes deep,
A melody where shadows sleep.

The forest listens, the stars reply,
A quiet bond between earth and sky.
And though their song is wild and free,
It carries a love for all to see.

Oh, wolves so bold, your hymn inspires,
A call of life through fierce desires.
For in your cry, the world will know,
A truth that lingers, a strength to grow.

171. The Star Maker

In the heavens, where silence reigns,
The star maker works, their hands unchained.
With strokes of light, they paint the skies,
A galaxy vast where dreams arise.

Each star they place, a beacon bright,
A tiny sun in endless night.
And though unseen by mortal eyes,
Their work endures in boundless skies.

Oh, maker wise, your art inspires,
A masterpiece through life's desires.
For in your stars, the heart will find,
A love that spans both space and time.

172. The Flame of the Hearth

The hearth it burns with a steady glow,

A warmth that all the world will know.
Its embers hum, its sparks they fly,
A gentle flame that will not die.

The home it guards, the hearts it keeps,
A quiet place where love still sleeps.
And though the nights grow long and cold,
Its fire burns, both bright and bold.

Oh, hearth so bright, your glow inspires,
A haven warm through life's desires.
For in your light, the world can see,
A love that shines eternally.

173. The Bridge of Stars

There lies a bridge the stars have spun,
A path of light where dreams are won.
Its arches gleam with silver glow,
A quiet road where spirits go.

The weary tread its shining span,
A journey vast, a soul's demand.
And though its course may seem unclear,
Its steps will lead to hearts sincere.

Oh, bridge of stars, your light inspires,
A guiding path through life's desires.
For in your span, the heart will find,
A bond that ties all humankind.

174. The Eternal Spring

The spring it flows with gentle grace,
Through rocks and roots, a sacred place.
Its waters clear, its song so light,

A melody through day and night.

It gives its life to fields and trees,
A gift of love the earth decrees.
And those who pause to drink its flow,
Will feel its truth, its ancient glow.

Oh, spring so pure, your heart inspires,
A source of life through deep desires.
For in your stream, the soul can see,
A timeless bond with eternity.

175. The Lonely Lighthouse

Upon the cliff where waves do roar,
The lighthouse stands on the rugged shore.
Its light it turns, its glow it sends,
A guiding hand where danger bends.

Its keeper walks the spiral stair,
A silent vigil, a sacred care.
And though the night is dark and vast,
Its golden beam will ever last.

Oh, lighthouse bright, your heart inspires,
A beacon bold through life's desires.
For in your glow, the world can see,
A love that guards eternity.

176. The Shadows of the Vale

In the vale where shadows fall,
The whispers rise, a haunting call.
Its trees they bow, its grasses sway,
A dance of dark where spirits play.

The wind it hums, the brook it sighs,
A melody beneath the skies.
And those who wander through its shade,

Will find the peace its whispers made.

Oh, shadowed vale, your grace inspires,
A quiet strength through life's desires.
For in your depths, the heart will see,
A beauty born of mystery.

177. The Flame of the Soul

A flame it burns within the heart,
A quiet force, a sacred spark.
Its light it glows, its warmth it gives,
A testament to all that lives.

The trials come, the storms may rise,
Yet still it shines beneath the skies.
And those who nurture its gentle glow,
Will find a strength they'll always know.

Oh, flame so bright, your truth inspires,
A fire bold through life's desires.
For in your light, the world can see,
A love that burns eternally.

178. The Mirror of the Lake

The lake it lies in tranquil peace,
A mirror bright where dreams release.
Its surface calm, its depths unknown,
A quiet realm the stars have sown.

The moon it casts its silver light,
A fleeting glow in the heart of night.
And those who gaze upon its face,
Will see their soul in its embrace.

Oh, lake so still, your beauty inspires,
A quiet joy through life's desires.
For in your depths, the heart will find,

A peace that lingers, unconfined.

179. The Song of the Mountains

The mountains hum in voices low,
A song of stone where rivers flow.
Their peaks they rise, their echoes sing,
A melody of everything.

The snow it falls, the rocks they stand,
A fortress vast, a timeless land.
And those who climb their towering heights,
Will find their soul in boundless flight.

Oh, mountains bold, your song inspires,
A hymn of earth through life's desires.
For in your peaks, the world can see,
A beauty born of majesty.

180. The Lantern Keeper

The keeper walks with lantern bright,
Through fields of dark, through endless night.
Its glow it casts a golden hue,
A guiding flame both old and new.

The shadows bend, the winds they wail,
Yet still they walk, they will not fail.
And those who follow where they lead,
Will find the strength their spirits need.

Oh, keeper bold, your light inspires,
A beacon true through life's desires.
For in your care, the heart will see,
A love that lasts eternally.

181. The Call of the Wild

The wild it calls in whispers fierce,

A voice that life and hearts will pierce.
Its rivers roar, its winds they cry,
A hymn of earth beneath the sky.

The trees they dance, the grasses sing,
A melody of boundless things.
And those who heed its mighty call,
Will find their truth within it all.

Oh, wild so vast, your voice inspires,
A force of life through fierce desires.
For in your call, the world will see,
A love that flows eternally.

182. The Weeping Rock

The rock it stands where waters fall,
A silent watcher through it all.
Its surface worn, its edges cracked,
A story told through time's impact.

The river carves its gentle face,
A quiet act of soft embrace.
And those who touch its weathered stone,
Will feel the life it's always known.

Oh, weeping rock, your grace inspires,
A steadfast love through life's desires.
For in your strength, the heart can see,
A beauty born of history.

183. The Stars' Lullaby

The stars they sing in voices bright,
A lullaby of endless night.
Their light it falls on earth below,
A gentle gift, a fleeting glow.

Their harmony it soothes the soul,

A melody that makes us whole.
And those who listen to their tune,
Will find a love beneath the moon.

Oh, stars so vast, your song inspires,
A tender hymn through life's desires.
For in your glow, the heart can see,
A truth that spans eternity.

184. The Bridge of Dreams

There lies a bridge that none can see,
A path that spans infinity.
Its arches built of hopes and fears,
A crossing bold through fleeting years.

The dreamers walk its fragile span,
Their steps a quest, their hearts a plan.
And though its path may twist and sway,
It leads to light beyond the gray.

Oh, bridge of dreams, your path inspires,
A journey vast through life's desires.
For in your steps, the world can find,
A truth that binds both heart and mind.

185. The Endless Road

The road it winds through hill and plain,
A timeless path through joy and pain.
Its stones are worn, its trail is clear,
A journey bold for hearts sincere.

The travelers walk with hopes untold,
Through skies of blue and sunsets gold.
And though the end may not be near,
Each step they take dissolves their fear.

Oh, endless road, your call inspires,
A quiet pull through life's desires.
For in your stretch, the heart will see,
A path to love and destiny.

186. The Whispering Wind

The wind it whispers soft and low,
A fleeting touch where shadows go.
It bends the trees, it stirs the grass,
A gentle hymn as seasons pass.

Its voice is light, its call is near,
A secret song for hearts to hear.
And though it fades, it leaves behind,
A quiet truth for heart and mind.

Oh, whispering wind, your song inspires,
A melody through life's desires.
For in your breath, the world can see,
A fleeting bond with eternity.

187. The Spirit of the Woods

The woods they hum with ancient grace,
A sacred song in shadowed space.
Their roots run deep, their branches high,
A temple vast beneath the sky.

The creatures move in quiet play,
A harmony through night and day.
And those who wander through its halls,
Will hear the tune that nature calls.

Oh, woods so vast, your heart inspires,
A hidden world through life's desires.
For in your shade, the soul will find,
A love that lingers, undefined.

188. The Guardian of the Shore

Upon the sands where waves do break,
A guardian stands for the ocean's sake.
Their watch is long, their eyes so clear,
A soul of strength that draws us near.

The tides they shift, the waters rise,
A force of life beneath the skies.
And though the storms may come and go,
The guardian's care will always show.

Oh, keeper bold, your watch inspires,
A steadfast love through life's desires.
For in your gaze, the world can see,
A bond with tides and eternity.

189. The Lantern of Night

The lantern glows through darkest skies,
A golden flame where silence lies.
Its light it casts a gentle hue,
A beacon bold, both old and new.

The shadows bow, the winds they wail,
But still it shines, it will not fail.
And those who follow where it leads,
Will find the strength their spirit needs.

Oh, lantern bright, your glow inspires,
A steady guide through life's desires.
For in your flame, the heart will see,
A path to hope and destiny.

190. The Meadow at Dawn

The meadow wakes with morning's light,
A golden field in soft delight.
Its grasses sway, its blossoms bloom,

A fragrant song of life's perfume.

The dew it glistens, the breeze it hums,
A quiet joy as day becomes.
And those who walk its tender ground,
Will feel the peace its heart has found.

Oh, meadow bright, your grace inspires,
A haven pure through life's desires.
For in your fields, the soul can see,
A harmony with eternity.

191. The Call of the Horizon

The horizon calls in tones so clear,
A beckoning voice for hearts sincere.
Its line it bends, its skies unfold,
A dream of blue and threads of gold.

The seas they stretch, the mountains rise,
A boundless world beneath the skies.
And those who chase its fleeting glow,
Will find the truths they long to know.

Oh, horizon wide, your voice inspires,
A boundless hope through life's desires.
For in your reach, the heart will find,
A journey bold through space and time.

192. The Keeper of Secrets

In shadowed halls where whispers grow,
The keeper guards what none may know.
Their hands are firm, their eyes are kind,
A quiet strength, a thoughtful mind.

The secrets held are not their own,
But truths of worlds that time has shown.
And though unseen, their work remains,

A sacred care through life's refrains.

Oh, keeper wise, your care inspires,
A quiet love through life's desires.
For in your hands, the heart will see,
A trust that spans eternity.

193. The Dance of the Stars

The stars they dance in heaven's dome,
A boundless waltz, a cosmic home.
Their light it flickers, faint yet strong,
A fleeting tune, a silent song.

The galaxies spin, the planets sway,
A rhythm vast that guides the way.
And those who gaze upon their glow,
Will find a love the stars bestow.

Oh, stars so bright, your dance inspires,
A harmony through life's desires.
For in your light, the world can see,
A boundless grace in mystery.

194. The Frozen River

The river sleeps beneath the ice,
A silent world, a sacrifice.
Its currents pause, its waters still,
A quiet rest through winter's chill.

The frost it gleams, the snow it falls,
A crystal cloak where silence calls.
And though it slumbers cold and deep,
Its heart still beats, it will not sleep.

Oh, frozen stream, your calm inspires,
A gentle rest through life's desires.
For in your peace, the soul can see,

A strength that flows eternally.

195. The Lighthouse Keeper's Song

The keeper hums a quiet tune,
Beneath the stars and watchful moon.
Their light it turns, their flame it glows,
A guiding hand where darkness flows.

The waves they crash, the winds they wail,
But still the keeper's care won't fail.
And those who sail through stormy seas,
Will find their hearts in gentle ease.

Oh, keeper bold, your song inspires,
A steadfast love through life's desires.
For in your care, the world can see,
A beacon strong for eternity.

196. The Eternal Flame

The eternal flame burns soft and bright,
A steady glow in endless night.
Its warmth it gives, its light it shares,
A quiet love that always cares.

The shadows fade, the cold retreats,
A tender glow where hearts may meet.
And though its fire may one day wane,
Its spirit lingers, free from pain.

Oh, flame so pure, your glow inspires,
A beacon strong through life's desires.
For in your light, the soul can see,
A love that burns eternally.

197. The Valley of Stars

Beneath the sky where the heavens gleam,
A valley rests in a starlit dream.
Its grasses sway in silver light,
A peaceful world in the heart of night.

The whispers rise from the earth below,
A melody soft, a gentle flow.
And those who tread this sacred land,
Will feel its touch, a guiding hand.

Oh, valley bright, your grace inspires,
A quiet calm through life's desires.
For in your glow, the heart will find,
A beauty vast, a peace unlined.

198. The Keeper of Time

The keeper stands with quiet grace,
Their eyes on time's unyielding pace.
Each tick and tock, each fleeting breath,
A testament to life and death.

Their hands they turn, their care is deep,
A guardian bold where moments sleep.
And though unseen, their work remains,
A thread that binds life's joys and pains.

Oh, keeper wise, your craft inspires,
A steady hand through life's desires.
For in your care, the world can see,
A harmony with eternity.

199. The Snow-Covered Peak

The mountain stands in winter's hold,
Its summit wrapped in icy gold.
The snow it glows, the frost it gleams,

A frozen world of timeless dreams.

Its cliffs are sharp, its winds they cry,
A fortress bold against the sky.
And those who climb its rugged face,
Will find their hearts in nature's grace.

Oh, mountain tall, your strength inspires,
A steady rise through life's desires.
For in your heights, the soul can see,
A beauty born of majesty.

200. The Lantern Bearer

Through forest deep and shadowed land,
The bearer walks with light in hand.
Their lantern glows, its flame it sways,
A guiding star through night's long maze.

The darkness bends, the path unfolds,
A quiet strength their heart upholds.
And those who follow where they lead,
Will find the light their spirits need.

Oh, bearer bright, your glow inspires,
A guiding hand through life's desires.
For in your light, the heart will see,
A path to hope and destiny.

201. The Moonlit River

The river shines in moonlight's glow,
A silver path where waters flow.
Its voice is soft, its ripples small,
A quiet hymn that touches all.

The stars they glimmer in its face,
A fleeting bond, a soft embrace.
And those who pause beside its stream,

Will find their hearts begin to dream.

Oh, river bright, your grace inspires,
A tranquil song through life's desires.
For in your flow, the soul can see,
A timeless bond with mystery.

202. The Bridge Beneath the Sky

The bridge it spans the endless blue,
A path of stone both old and new.
Its arches strong, its journey clear,
A crossing built for hearts sincere.

The travelers walk with steps of grace,
Their dreams reflected in its face.
And though its stones may wear with time,
Its strength endures, its soul sublime.

Oh, bridge so bold, your form inspires,
A lasting hope through life's desires.
For in your span, the heart will find,
A path that ties all humankind.

203. The Forest's Lullaby

The forest hums with a tender tune,
A lullaby beneath the moon.
Its leaves they rustle, its roots they sing,
A melody of everything.

The night it falls, the shadows rise,
A quiet peace beneath the skies.
And those who rest within its arms,
Will find their hearts in nature's charms.

Oh, forest deep, your song inspires,
A soothing hymn through life's desires.
For in your shade, the soul can see,

A beauty born of unity.

204. The Whisper of the Tides

The tides they whisper soft and low,
A rhythmic song where waters flow.
Their currents pull, their waves they bend,
A cycle vast without an end.

The shore it listens, the rocks they sigh,
A harmony beneath the sky.
And those who feel the ocean's call,
Will find its love within it all.

Oh, tides so vast, your voice inspires,
A gentle flow through life's desires.
For in your song, the world can see,
A truth that flows eternally.

205. The Midnight Bell

The bell it tolls at midnight's hour,
A solemn chime of quiet power.
Its echo rolls through darkened air,
A whispered hope, a gentle prayer.

The stars they listen, the moon it glows,
A fleeting calm the bell bestows.
And those who hear its steady ring,
Will find the peace its tones can bring.

Oh, midnight bell, your sound inspires,
A fleeting joy through life's desires.
For in your chime, the heart will see,
A beauty found in mystery.

206. The Path Through Shadows

The path it winds through shadowed lands,

A quiet trail through time's demands.
Its stones are worn, its turns are steep,
A road where secrets softly sleep.

The trees they guard, their branches sway,
A solemn watch through night and day.
And those who tread its hidden way,
Will find their hearts no longer stray.

Oh, shadowed path, your course inspires,
A quiet walk through life's desires.
For in your steps, the soul will see,
A bond with time and destiny.

207. The Golden Horizon

The horizon glows with hues of fire,
A canvas bright, a world's desire.
Its line it bends, its colors blend,
A fleeting art that knows no end.

The sun it sets, the stars arise,
A quiet dance through endless skies.
And those who gaze upon its glow,
Will find the truths they long to know.

Oh, horizon wide, your light inspires,
A fleeting hope through life's desires.
For in your glow, the heart will see,
A beauty born of eternity.

Here is another **20 long, lyrical poems** to keep this beautiful collection growing. Each one is crafted to inspire and resonate deeply. □

208. The Song of the Morning

The morning sings with gentle light,
A melody to end the night.
Its voice it rises, soft and clear,
A quiet call for hearts to hear.

The dew it clings to blades of grass,
A fleeting touch as moments pass.
And those who wake to greet the day,
Will find their dreams not far away.

Oh, morning bright, your song inspires,
A hymn of hope through life's desires.
For in your glow, the world can see,
A path to love and harmony.

209. The Watcher of the Waves

Upon the cliff where oceans roar,
The watcher stands to guard the shore.
Their gaze is fixed on waters wide,
A steady soul through time and tide.

The waves they crash, the winds they wail,
Yet still they stand, they will not fail.
And those who see their quiet grace,
Will find their fears begin to erase.

Oh, watcher bold, your strength inspires,
A steadfast heart through life's desires.
For in your care, the world can see,
A love that guards eternity.

210. The Meadow's Glow

The meadow glows in sunset's hue,
A golden light through skies of blue.
Its grasses sway, its blossoms shine,

A fleeting glimpse of the divine.

The shadows stretch, the day grows still,
A moment rare, a breath to fill.
And those who pause within its space,
Will feel the earth's enduring grace.

Oh, meadow bright, your beauty inspires,
A haven pure through life's desires.
For in your glow, the heart will see,
A harmony with eternity.

211. The Keeper of Stars

The keeper walks through skies so vast,
Where stars are born and echoes cast.
Their hands they weave the threads of light,
A quiet art through endless night.

The constellations bow and turn,
A cosmic map for hearts that yearn.
And those who gaze upon their skies,
Will find their soul begins to rise.

Oh, keeper wise, your work inspires,
A universe through life's desires.
For in your stars, the heart will see,
A boundless truth, a mystery.

212. The River of Dreams

The river flows with dreams untold,
Its waters bright, its current bold.
It carries hopes through night and day,
A quiet guide along the way.

Its ripples sing, its depths they gleam,
A fleeting path, a living dream.
And those who follow where it leads,

Will find the love their spirit needs.

Oh, river vast, your song inspires,
A quiet truth through life's desires.
For in your flow, the heart will see,
A timeless bond with destiny.

213. The Silent Forest

The forest rests in twilight's glow,
A quiet realm where spirits go.
Its trees they stand, their roots they weave,
A sacred bond that none perceive.

The winds they hush, the leaves they sigh,
A melody beneath the sky.
And those who wander through its halls,
Will hear the voice that nature calls.

Oh, forest deep, your grace inspires,
A tranquil space through life's desires.
For in your stillness, the heart will see,
A beauty born of unity.

214. The Echo of the Hills

The hills they hum with echoes past,
A timeless song that will not last.
Their voices rise, their whispers play,
A melody of yesterday.

The grasses bow, the stones they sing,
A quiet tune of everything.
And those who stand upon their crest,
Will find their hearts begin to rest.

Oh, hills so wide, your echoes inspire,
A quiet hymn through life's desires.
For in your sound, the world can see,

A harmony with history.

215. The Moonlit Harbor

The harbor sleeps in moonlight's glow,
A silver calm where waters flow.
The ships they rest, their sails unwind,
A fleeting peace for heart and mind.

The stars they glimmer, soft and bright,
A tender guide through endless night.
And those who linger by its shore,
Will find the dreams they longed for.

Oh, harbor kind, your peace inspires,
A haven sweet through life's desires.
For in your stillness, the heart will see,
A love that flows eternally.

216. The Spirit of the Flame

The flame it burns with steady light,
A force of warmth in endless night.
Its flickers dance, its glow it hums,
A quiet hymn for all it comes.

The shadows bow, the darkness fades,
A fleeting truth its fire conveys.
And those who nurture its tender glow,
Will find the strength they long to know.

Oh, flame so bright, your fire inspires,
A guiding warmth through life's desires.
For in your light, the heart can see,
A strength that burns eternally.

217. The Desert's Lament

The desert sings in whispers low,

A solemn tune where few will go.
Its sands they shift, its winds they sigh,
A haunting hymn beneath the sky.

The sun it burns, the shadows grow,
A quiet truth the desert knows.
And those who tread its endless plain,
Will find its beauty through its pain.

Oh, desert vast, your voice inspires,
A quiet strength through life's desires.
For in your sands, the soul will see,
A love that lasts eternally.

218. The Frozen Meadow

The meadow sleeps beneath the frost,
Its beauty stilled, its whispers lost.
Its grasses gleam in winter's glow,
A quiet world of ice and snow.

The trees they stand in silent grace,
A crystal touch on nature's face.
And those who pause within its space,
Will feel the peace that time can't erase.

Oh, meadow cold, your heart inspires,
A beauty pure through life's desires.
For in your stillness, the world can see,
A timeless love, a mystery.